OH, SO SWEET TO LIVE SUGAR FREE

Five Success Strategies to Eliminate the Progression to Diabetes

KATHY "SUGAR FREE GIRL "WILLIAMS

Williams Consulting Group, LLC
Maryland

Oh, So Sweet to Live Sugar Free
Five Success Strategies to Eliminate the Progression to Diabetes

Williams Consulting Group, LLC.
Clarksburg, MD

Special discounts are available on bulk quantity discount purchase by book clubs, associations and special interest groups. For details email: info@ilivesugarfree.com.

Book Edited by Sharon Arredondo
Photography by Christopher Culotta

ISBN: 978-1-7336572-0-4 (print)
ISBN: 978-1-7336572-1-1 (eBook)

To my loving supportive husband, Bernard, my rock,
for making everything possible.

To my parents, Francis and Doris Wansley,
for raising me to believe that anything is possible.

To my children, Justice, Karen and Joseph,
for seeing new possibilities.

Contents

A NOTE FROM THE AUTHOR

Winning my own personal battle over a diagnosis that would seem hopeless to many became the motivation to write this book. When told I was pre-diabetic, I could have accepted it and followed a pre-destined path based on medical studies. Instead, I chose to discover a healthy option for eliminating the progression to diabetes and I am now ready to share my success so others can experience the same victory.

The statistics are stunning:
- A CDC study published in 2014 noted that 29 million persons in the U.S. had diabetes.
- 86 million people are classified as having pre-diabetes—nearly a third of the U.S. adult population.
- Diabetes remains the 7th leading cause of death in the United States in 2015.
- According to the Centers for Disease Control and Prevention, nearly 1 in 10 women develop gestational diabetes during pregnancy,
  - Women with a history of gestational diabetes are estimated to have seven times the risk of developing diabetes, compared with women who didn't have gestational diabetes.

I'm in the diabetes prevention business! I don't want anyone to have to suffer from something so pervasive and preventable. Just because you are diagnosed with gestational or pre-diabetes does not mean that you have to progress to the disease.

INTRODUCTION

There are many people in life who dream of finding some magical formula for healthy living. Waking up every morning full of energy and ready to face the day. Less aches and pains, less inflammation, and more motivation to embark on "bucket-list" adventures or just living a full healthy life.

You may say, "I'm not that type of person." However, if we did not desire those kinds of experiences then Hollywood would not be successful creating hit movies that show people living those kinds of lives.

The way we feel has an incredible impact on what we do. For many, it is difficult to move beyond the basic responsibilities of our job or home before exhaustion settles in and dictates the remainder of the day. There is a way to feel more energetic and more alive and it is possible to capture those moments that make life worth living. Running, swimming, playing with your children or grandchildren can be fun again. Hiking, hunting, fishing, bicycling, or some other favorite activity can be something you look forward to again.

What kind of a solution can solve a problem that seems to be an epidemic of proportion? Amazingly enough, the problem solver is also the key to helping diabetics move forward with less dependency on unnatural resources. In fact, this solution can even prevent those who are pre-diabetic from ever crossing the line over into a life with diabetes.

The answer for a more abundant life that is lengthened in years is not the fountain of youth. You have the power to solve this problem by making the right choices and changing what is considered "the norm" for regular consumption. It all starts with sugar free living. Believe me, it's *"So Sweet to Live Sugar Free."* Follow me on this journey as I share the steps that changed my life forever!

CHAPTER 1

Step #1: It's Decision Time

When I started the journey of becoming sugar-free it was a decision process for me. Every road to success must begin with an unmovable, steadfast decision. You must be like a tree that is planted by the water and is not easily moved.

The motivation for my decisive action began with my pre-diabetes diagnosis. I looked at what I wanted; a long happy life and especially wanted no part of injecting myself with insulin. I did not want diabetes and all the inconveniences and health risks that come along with that lifestyle. Being in the medical field for over 20 years; I know diabetes is a systemic disease affecting circulation, eyesight, wound healing, your heart and more. All these effects are systemic, progressive and chronic. Nor did I desire to have my family and friends concerned about my health or wondering if I would be around to see them accomplish their life goals. When I put things into perspective, the decision was easy.

What I want is a long healthy life! I want to be here for my children, grandchildren and great-grandchildren. Beyond the longing to be here for those who love me and depend on me, I also want to achieve more for myself. I love to travel, meet people and especially help others. Experiencing new adventures with my husband and family without the hindrances of health concerns is one of my goals.

There are those who suffer severely from diabetes and the outcome can be devastating. Physical conditions that develop over time leave individuals unable to get around on their own because of nerve damage, wound healing and even heart disease. I am determined to maintain the power over my independence. This determination was not fueling a short-term goal but driving me to make a life change that would enable me to stay on the course for as long as I live.

You are probably asking what made me get tested. Well I knew the major signs of diabetes are excessive thirst, frequent urination and fatigue. Being in the healthcare field for several years, I self-diagnosed often and often explained away things that should have driven me to the doctor. In my case, I am orthostatic which means if I do not eat or drink, I pass out. That said, I drink water constantly and therefore since I have three kids all I have to do is stand up and I am running to the bathroom (literally). I'm also a "Type A" personality so I am constantly on the go. You guessed it! Since I am "on" 24/7; I sit down to watch a show at 8 p.m. or 9 p.m. and the show ends up watching me. I told you I could explain things away! I'm always in the bathroom and was tired, but for good reason. The dry mouth I could not explain. I would wake up in the middle of the night or first thing in the morning with "cotton mouth" (excessive thirst on steroids!). Thirst that was not quenched by a few sips of water, but an entire bottle of water.

Hence, I made an appointment for a physical, explained my symptoms and based on the symptoms; my doctor scheduled a fasting glucose test. The diagnosis was Pre-Diabetes!

As a healthcare professional, I acted on this diagnosis. Mind you it took me a minute, two months to be exact, before I scheduled my appointment with the nutritionist. My journey began after my first visit. The reason I acted was because of my family history and the fact that I have seen first hand the damaging systemic effects of diabetes especially as you age. There is a definitive link between diabetes and heart disease. Guess what runs in my family? Diabetes and heart disease.

Ten years prior to my diagnosis my twin sister, Karen, was diagnosed as being pre-diabetic. She too gave up sugar, but she gave it up "cold turkey". She did such a good job that she was out hiking and passed out because she became hypoglycemic (low blood sugar). She has since introduced sugar back into her life but does so sparingly. My mom was truly my muse. About seven years ago, she too was diagnosed with pre-diabetes and sought help by attending a yearlong pre-diabetes class at the YMCA. The YMCA program concentrated on diet and exercise and was based on the Diabetes Prevention Program Group Lifestyle Balance ™

(DPP GLB) (The program I would later be certified in). The program is based on a balanced lifestyle approach to diet (counting fat grams) and exercise. She was the only one in her class that just followed the diet component; but still reached her goals. At the end of the program, she was successful in reducing her weight by seven percent, HA1c to a normal level, blood pressure, and cholesterol. Unfortunately, she too has re-introduced sugar into her life. But I am convinced, that when they make the decision to follow my system, they will have the lifelong effects I have. In chapter 6, you will find the secret to my long-term sustained success. The powerful game changer!

Do you see the pattern? It was right in front of my face and I did not act until I started having symptoms and was diagnosed. Later in chapter 7, you will see how I struggled and fought constantly with this process. But you can see that with this knowledge from my family history and my medical history, there were things that I just could not ignore.

It is easy for people to focus on what they don't have and to allow their thoughts to be saturated with negative thinking. This can lead to grave disappointment and regrets. I am just the opposite! I am a glass half full girl! If I can think it, I can achieve it! Anything worth having (healthy living) is worth working for! Therefore, for me it all started with the decision to make a change.

Step 1: Decide
- Decide what you want and what you don't want…
  - I want a long healthy life.
  - I want a happy and FUN life filled with Joy and Peace!
  - I want to travel the world with my family.
  - I want to spend time with my kids, grandkids, great grandkids…
  - I want to help others live healthy lives without diabetes or heart disease.
  - I do not want diabetes.
  - I do not want to inject myself with insulin.
  - I do not want heart disease.

What do you want? What are you waiting for? What's getting in your way?

Write your short term goals:

_____
_____
_____
_____
_____
_____
_____
_____
_____
_____
_____
_____
_____
_____

Where do you want to be in 5, 10 years? What type of health do you want to enjoy? How do you want to feel 5 or 10 years from now? How do you want to feel in your retirement?

Write your long term goals:

_____
_____
_____
_____
_____
_____
_____
_____
_____
_____
_____
_____
_____

CHAPTER 2

Step #2: Seek Help

Making such a drastic lifestyle change didn't come easy. The first step was making a bold decision to change some of the most instinctive habits and to combat my deepest cravings. This was going to require activating step two; Getting Help!

When I was diagnosed with being pre-diabetic, my Hemoglobin A1c (HbA1c) level was 6.0. The doctor suggested that I visit a nutritionist. HbA1c level below 5.7 percent is considered normal; anywhere between 5.7 and 6.4 percent signals pre-diabetes. Type 2 diabetes is diagnosed when the HbA1c is over 6.5 percent. For many Type 2 diabetics, the goal is to lower HbA1c levels to a healthier level. I am sharing my story so that you can take the necessary steps to prevent the diagnosis. I did not heed the signs around me until I was diagnosed as being pre-diabetes. You don't have to wait.

I listened to the doctor's advice and scheduled an appointment with a nutritionist. Looking back, it's plain to see that the nutritionist had her own expectation of what our first encounter would be. When I met her, she shared that she expected to see a much larger lady. Most of the time, it is assumed that a pre-diabetic or diabetics are substantially overweight. However, I am 5'1" and at that time weighed 130 lbs. I wore a size 8 and didn't feel like I needed to lose weight. It's not uncommon to see a woman of my size described as "curvy". I have three beautiful kids, and as a result a "pouch" of a stomach.

Size and weight can be a great inspiration for some people to change their lifestyle when it comes to the foods and substances that they consume. However, this was not the motivation for me. It was the simple understanding that my diet needed to change if the quality and length of my days were going to be sustained. The fact that diabetes runs in my family swayed my thoughts on a new way of living. In the past, I have been successful in giving up sodas and sugar many times for the 40 days of Lent, but always went back.

This time, I had the motivation of the diagnosis to help me seek the support I needed from a nutritionist. I had not been successful making a permanent lifestyle change on my own at this point in my life. Why would I continue doing the same thing and hope for a better result? If you realize that the direction of your life will not lead to results you want, don't be afraid to seek help.

Some believe seeking help is a sign of weakness. Not me, I gladly ask for help if it means I can get better. Every great success is noted for the ability to change and overcome. Seek the help you need! Looking back, it is easy to see why I sought out coaches especially when I made lifestyle changes. It's not because we do not have access to the information; Google, Siri, books and even Dr. Oz. In this case, my nutritionist had a plan for me and held me accountable. As things progressed, I then further developed and refined my system. I have used coaches in business, fitness and now for my health. They also give me the kick in the pants I need to stay on track and make bold moves necessary for my long term success.

Step 1: Decide
Step 2: Seek Help
- I sought help to support my decision.
- I knew I could not do it alone without the guidance and expertise of my nutritionist.
- My nutritionist was just one of the coaches that motivated me and held me accountable to my new lifestyle.

How many times have you started and stopped? What makes you think you can do it on your own? Are you willing to seek help?

_____

_____

_____

_____

_____

_____

_____

_____

_____

_____

_____

_____

_____

_____

CHAPTER 3

Drink This! Not That!

Some moments in life make an indelible mark on the timeline of your memories. I can remember the diagnosis of being pre-diabetic like it was yesterday. November of 2015, became a defining moment that would forever change the way I viewed sugar.

I went to the nutritionist in January of 2016 and was told in no uncertain terms that I needed to give up sugar. For some people this kind of information can be frightening, especially those who have a persistent sweet tooth. Although I initially didn't want to fully accept the recommendation of "no sugar," it was not a concept that seemed unrealistic.

Mainly due to my upbringing, I'm not the type of person who craves a dessert at the end of every meal. When I was growing up, my mom was always on a diet. We didn't have Kool-Aid or sodas in the house nor was it mandatory to have a piece of cake or pie for dessert.

Our cake and ice cream experiences usually revolved around someone having a birthday or some other special celebration. I didn't necessarily have a background that led to eating sweets all the time.

When I met with the nutritionist, we had four sessions. During the first session, we talked about my diet through a series of questions. We walked through what I ate, what I drank, what times of the day this took place and anything that revolved around my sugar intake.

The nutritionist looked at me and said, "Kathy, you need to give up sugar." You would think that settled the issue, but that was not the case. I went back and forth with her for about three or four minutes as I tried to divulge my wealth of knowledge. I tried to convince her that I didn't eat a lot of sugar. I told her, "I thought all you had to do was eat a protein when you ate sweets for your body to process the sugar appropriately." Of course, I explained all this to her, but she was steadfast in her recommendation. So, I took it to heart and the journey began.

Only a month after meeting with the nutritionist, my first test was a business trip to Switzerland! Chocolate Capital of the WORLD! How did I do it? It was not easy. I made the decision and stuck with it. I maintained my commitment to myself and put things in the context of trade-offs. Was this dessert worth an insulin needle to my stomach?

But what I realized, as I investigated my diet, was that most of my calories were from my drink choices. Don't get me wrong, I adore chocolate, cake, sweet potato pie, Oreo's, chocolate shakes, ice cream, cookies and especially caramel! I also loved to snack when my kids snacked, so it wasn't uncommon to eat sweets on a regular basis.

I may not have had drinks loaded with sugar in my childhood, but as I ventured out on my own, it didn't take long to fall prey to the habit. Much of the common drinks available today have more sugar per serving than is often realized.

I had to make some changes. A typical day might look like this: I would get the day started with either orange juice or hot chocolate. At lunch, I would have a Pepsi and every now and then a Pepsi at dinner (especially when I ate crabs, pizza or wings). I didn't keep sodas in the house, but they were a convenient drink when I was out and about. I also drank soda when I traveled and when in all day meetings or conferences.

I never acquired the taste for coffee so, in order to take sugar out of my diet, I discovered cappuccino. I replaced the hot chocolate in the morning with a cappuccino sweetened with Stevia and stopped drinking regular sodas. Quitting sodas cold turkey was a huge challenge for me. I made the switch from regular sodas to diet soda. I'll share my process of eliminating sodas from my life in the Gradual Replacement (Chapter 5).

Please believe me when I say going through this process is still a work in progress. The important thing is that you keep going. Part of eliminating sugar from my diet was to eliminate all sweets. However, I had to overcome my own concerns during this process. For instance, I know that some artificial sweeteners have been linked to cancer. Therefore, having regular sodas instead of diet sodas became an excuse for me to remain where I was comfortable.

Once the decision was made to do whatever was necessary to make a change, I was convinced that a temporary switch from regular sodas to diet sodas was worth the risk. The key to increasing my return on this risk was to press on toward removing all sodas from my daily beverage choices. The right mindset paid off. The diet soda excursion was very short-lived. It only lasted about six months before I stopped drinking diet sodas and then moved to unsweetened iced tea sweetened with Stevia. The transition was from a regular Pepsi to a diet Pepsi then to no sodas at all and eventually just drinking water, milk and unsweetened iced tea and replacing my hot chocolate with a cappuccino. This is what I like to call a gradual transition or "step down process".

After having success with these life altering adjustments, I found there were other beverage options that would work for me. I transitioned to preferring flavored sparkling water which added some flavor instead of only having plain water. I also made changes in my alcoholic preferences.

Drinking wine with my husband at dinner is now a thing of the past. If you do choose to drink, there are spiked seltzer beverages with zero to five (5) grams of sugar. (I have listed the brands in Appendix 1). Alternately, fruit infused vodka and club soda is a low sugar substitute as well.

Since progressing through this process, I have learned how to have these items in my house and not be tempted. The reason is that I have gradually made these life changing substitutions. I am modeling behavior for my kids, my kids are by no means living sugar free. YET!

Drink This! Not That!

- Eliminate sodas by choosing unsweetened iced tea and flavored sparkling water. (See Appendix 5 for a list of brands)
- Replace your hot chocolate with cappuccino sweetened with Stevia.
- Eliminate all juices and replace them with the whole fruit.
- If you choose to drink alcohol, try spiked sparkling waters as an alternative to wine.(See Appendix 1 for the list of brands).

What small drink changes can you commit to this week?

Write your weekly commitments:

_____
_____
_____
_____
_____
_____
_____
_____
_____
_____
_____
_____
_____
_____

CHAPTER 4

Eat This! Not That!

My first visit to the nutritionist certainly greeted me with many surprises from her initial assessment of my appearance to her final diagnosis. My second visit with her was the key to moving forward with this sugar free expedition. We walked through her recommendations for my diet step-by-step.

The nutritionist gave me a meal plan for breakfast, lunch and dinner. She also added suggestions for two snacks in addition to the meals. All of this was based on a percent of fat, cholesterol and protein that I could eat during the day. After meeting with her, I began to look at my meal planning differently. This would affect the way I eat out and how I shop for groceries.

The third session I had with my nutritionist was not a regular office visit. This meeting was scheduled by phone and the discussion dealt with actions that could help me better assess what changes were needed. I was shown the importance of keeping a record of what I was eating. Sometimes, we don't realize how often we slip up or have something "small" that makes a "big" difference.

When you record what you are doing, you don't have to depend on your memory to help you recall the details. The use of apps like "Apple's Activity" "Fitbit", "My Fitness Pal", "My Plate" and "HealthTrac" take the guessing out of monitoring fat and sugar grams. With all the distractions that take place in a single day, it's hard to remember, what you ate. For example, to recall what you ate today may be simple, but the amount of sugar you ate over the past three days, now that's a different story. Remembering every item you've eaten, and the portion size can be a daunting task if you don't write it down. The nutritionist helped me work on doing a journal of what I was eating.

Simply seeing a list of items eaten on a piece of paper can be revealing. Going through the process of thinking about each item you ingested and how much sugar was in it can be eye opening. The power of this process makes the effort and discipline to follow through totally worth it.

Three sessions with the nutritionist taught me a lot and had me viewing life from a new perspective. The paradigm shift that was required was enough to be overwhelming if I would have taken it in all at once. Thankfully, this was a process that unfolded along the way making each forward progression a reachable goal.

There was one final session where we went over the importance of looking at labels. Yes, it is necessary to look at labels. The process may add some time to your shopping, but it is also adding time to your life. The nutritionist's recommendation for my daily consumption was 47% carbohydrates, 29% fat and 24% from protein and if I consumed sugar, less than five grams. You can even have moderate amounts of alcohol. However, even "heart-healthy red wine" breaks down to sugar.

Recommended low sugar proteins:	Recommended low sugar grains:
• Low-Fat Dairy (Milk, Cheese, Yogurt) • Eggs • Nuts • Fish • Shellfish • Beef • Pork	• Whole-Grain Breads • Whole-Grain Pasta • Brown Rice • Oatmeal

Recommended low sugar fruits and vegetables:

• All Berries	• Kiwi
• Broccoli	• Cauliflower
• Kale	• Bok Choy
• Cabbage	• Brussels Sprouts
• Mushrooms	• Tomatoes
• Radishes	• All Leafy Green Vegetables

I took things a step further and researched high glycemic index foods to eliminate from my diet. According to Accredited Practicing Dietitian (APD) Sonya Stanley, "The Glycemic Index (GI) ranks foods according to how quickly they are digested. Low GI foods are slowly digested and therefore more filling, which can be beneficial for healthy weight and blood glucose levels."

Looking at the labels on the food you consume is helpful for measuring, but just because you see a low-GI label on your food doesn't make the selected food healthy. Discovering foods that are truly low-GI will help your diet greatly.
- Legumes like kidney beans, baked beans and chickpeas
- Sweet potato
- Low-fat dairy products including milk and yogurt
- Whole fruits in general such as apples and oranges
- Nuts
- Pasta not the quick cook varieties
- Wholegrain breads and cereals
- Oats
- Brown Rice
- Water (it's best for water to always be your first choice of beverage)

Remember big changes often require due diligence as you persist through a process. For me the first step was a decision, the second step was to seek help, but it didn't stop there. Step three required me to do my own research. That's when I started to investigate both the elimination of sugar and understanding the difference between choosing low glycemic foods and eliminating high glycemic index foods.

Once I knew what foods were high in sugar and which foods had low-GI levels then I understood what I needed to take out of my life. For example, I stopped eating bananas and now eat kiwi for potassium. In some cultures, it is common to have rice at every meal. That was not something I had to have regularly, but the starch we had frequently at our meals was corn. You can probably guess that corn was another high-GI food, so I put a stop to eating corn. (Appendix 2 outlines a list of the Low, Medium and High glycemic foods)

Making major changes doesn't always mean eliminating everything. I now watch and reduce my carbohydrate intake as well. I enjoy eating pancakes, but I do have to make partial sacrifices. For me, a partial sacrifice was to have pancakes occasionally but no longer put syrup on them. Instead of having a stack of two or three pancakes, now I have half of one with no syrup.

Be careful with items you select that say, "No sugar added", because they may contain another form or sugar (dextrose, fructose, corn syrup, etc.).

Quitting anything abruptly can lead to short lived results. When you quit something cold turkey, your body does nothing but crave it. Success comes when you ease into your new choices and step down gradually from old routines. My purpose for writing this book is to share my success strategies.

Step 1: Decide
Step 2: Seek Help
Step 3: Research
- I researched and discovered that high glycemic index foods are just as damaging as sugar.
- I eliminated banana, pineapple, corn and have reduced the amounts of white potatoes and pasta I consume.
    - I replaced bananas with kiwi for potassium and vitamin C.
    - I have eliminated corn and have reduced the amounts of rice and pasta.
    - I have also replaced white potatoes with sweet potatoes.

**What do you know about glycemic index foods?
See Appendix 2 for an abbreviated list.**

After reviewing Appendix 2, what high glycemic index foods could you replace or eliminate?

_____

_____

_____

_____

_____

_____

_____

_____

_____

_____

_____

_____

_____

CHAPTER 5

Step #3: Research and Gradual Replacement

My walk was not immediate and by no means cold turkey…it was a process. After I decided, I sought the help of a nutritionist and then I researched.

When I researched, I not only learned about the glycemic index, I also had to educate myself with the language of diabetes. (Appendix 3 outlines key terms you will hear from your doctor).

Next, I measured! I did this to understand how, what I ate affected my body and blood sugar levels. I started to gradually replace things that were not good for my system. I now choose what's best for my health and still have the flavor in my life.

I started by removing sugar from my diet; that meant sweets. I changed from having a Pepsi a day at lunch to going to diet soda. And again, my belief was that the artificial sweeteners cause cancer and even though I knew they were bad for me that was my gradual step down from cane sugar.

Six months of consuming artificial sweeteners was not the right choice or direction for me long term because of my family's history of cancer. At this point, I drink water (sparkling or still), milk and unsweet iced tea with Stevia. Water should always be your first beverage choice. I drink eight to ten glasses or at least four bottles of water a day. This keeps me hydrated, full and of course running to the bathroom! You can also infuse fruit into your water. Lemon, mint or cucumber are refreshing quick and easy ways to add flavor without calories.

Other gradual changes included how to handle "that time of the month". There are sugar free chocolates, cakes, cookies and candy options that I ate during the first six months when I was drinking diet sodas. I do not recommend the ones sweetened with the chemical sweeteners as there are now more and more Stevia sweetened options.

I've stopped eating the sugar free chocolate, cakes, candy and cookies. My latest find is Planter's cocoa covered almonds! 24 of them are just three grams of sugar! They assist my sweet tooth during my 2 p.m. need for a pick me up and satisfy my craving for chocolate during "that time of the month". Of course, almonds are good for you so I keep a jar at my desk, in my pantry and have them daily. My kids finally tasted them and now have them in their lunch. The key is to have alternatives on hand.

What else was gradual for me? I would say the other gradual thing for me was alcohol. I'm not a drinker per se; I drank socially and would have a glass of wine with my husband at dinner. But over time, I've seen that if I have a drink with dinner my sugar level is still high in the morning. Thus, I eliminated wine.

Eat This! Not That!
- Switch to oatmeal with apple or pecans instead of banana.
- Reduce your carbohydrate intake by eliminating buns or breads.
  - Have a lettuce wrapped burger and eat a few fries. It may be just me, given the choice of a bun or fries. I'll choose the fries all day!
- Substitute oranges for orange juice.
  - I no longer drink juices and now only eat the raw fruit.
- Need potassium? Try kiwi instead of banana. Kiwi are also high in vitamin A, vitamin C and calcium.
- Add protein powder to fruit smoothies to offset the amount of sugar in the fruit.

What questions do you have for your next doctor's appointment?

Take a few notes:

_____
_____
_____
_____
_____
_____
_____
_____
_____
_____
_____
_____
_____
_____

CHAPTER 6

Step #4: Measuring Required

Decide first, seek help and then do as I did and start your own research. I started by eliminating the sugar at the onset of my newfound regimen. Then I investigated high glycemic index foods and removed those from my diet, not all at once, but as I learned about them. It's easy to stop your forward progression if you only have a short-term goal to achieve, but I set many markers along the way. My ultimate destination: No longer being diagnosed a Pre-Diabetic! This demanded that I remain persistent in looking for other ways to remove calories from the sugar source perspective like alcohol and soda.

One of the other keys that unlocked the door to the success I achieved was measurement. I don't think a lot of people think about the importance of measurement as a pre-diabetic.

Very early on I had a conversation, probably a year into my transformation, with a colleague who had lost about 30 pounds. I asked him how he did it and he shared that he did the ever-popular Atkins Diet. I shared what was going on with me and how I was trying to make a difference by radically changing my eating and drinking choices. Then he shared something that opened my eyes like a magician sharing how he had performed a trick. This one secret became a critical step for me. Primarily because I am a data person and I know for a fact that to have a proper outcome you must first understand what's going on in your body.

Diet plans and nutritional strategies generally work for everyone across the board, but we all must learn how our individual body responds to certain foods and drink. There may be something that doesn't seem like it would have much influence on your sugar levels, but the impact could be greater than you realize.

My colleague shared how he got a glucose meter to take his blood sugar levels every day when he woke up in the morning. He would also check his levels just before and then two hours after a snack or meal. This helps you to fully understand where sugars may be slipping into your system. Although you may be taking things out of your diet and cutting back on carbs, there could still be foods that increase your levels. Determine what food is sabotaging your efforts. **Measure!**

When you choose to eat or drink something and then measure your glucose levels to see how your body responds, your understanding greatly motivates you to make better choices. This is the reason why I eliminated wine from my diet and only occasionally drink spiked seltzer water. In the evening after dinner, my husband and I would sit down to watch a movie or just relax and I would have popcorn and some wine. The next day, I would find that my blood sugar would be sky high. This is the reason this step is so critical, without this data feedback loop, I would not have a mechanism to determine what food or drink and what amount are affecting my overall health.

Imagine yourself in this scenario. I've done well throughout the course of the day, but as the conclusion of my daily routine draws near, one simple choice wreck my progress. The combination of the time of day and the fact that there is a high sugar content in wine, basically breaks down to having a bowl of sugar before I went to bed.

The only way I could have known how much my routine for relaxation was working against me was to measure. This is the cornerstone of my personal program. **You cannot monitor what you don't measure.** If you measure early on and understand that when you eat three pancakes and an omelet it leads to having high blood sugar, then you can make immediate adjustments. It does not necessarily mean, "No more pancakes for you." Maybe you cut back to one pancake instead of the stack of three. I now eat a half of a pancake without syrup, with a protein, so I can enjoy my cappuccino!

When you measure and you track the results; like an experiment you will find how your body reacts to certain foods and/or the quantities of those foods you eat. Knowing what it is in your diet that creates the greatest dynamic alterations will help you make better choices. These are the better choices that lead to the longevity you first sought after. All the things you decided from the very beginning that you wanted could happen with the right consistent choices.

My colleague who was so helpful with the insight on measuring my blood sugar levels gave me a good example by sharing one of the changes he made. His mother-in-law made a delicious sauce that was more of a gravy substance put over noodles. This combination, as well as the quantity, would send his blood sugar through the roof. He was able to make the needed adjustment away from carbs by substituting traditional pasta for spaghetti squash. A bigger adjustment was needed still. The amount that he was eating also contributed to the outcome he faced. Therefore, he figured out what quantity would keep him satisfied without causing a spike in blood sugars. The upshot is powerful choices that he was only able to make because he measured the results of his consumption. These positive changes led to other positive choices such as exercising consistently. He also made the decision to add more protein to his meal choices. Remember it is not all about elimination.

The basis for what worked well for me was making the decision, getting help, doing my own research and measuring. You don't have to do all the research for yourself because I've already done this and sharing it with you allows you to get a quick start on your journey. I have the lists already prepared for you, so you can make better choices. The main component to my program is to measure. Knowledge is power.

You don't know what's going on in your body without seeing it. You cannot feel the difference in your system unless you are already diabetic. Some symptoms include frequent urination, excessive thirst or fatigue. Sometimes, those who have dealt with diabetes for a significant length of time have a sense of what they feel and what it means with their blood sugar levels. Ultimately the truth remains that you cannot monitor what you do not measure.

One of the reasons I desire to help others who deal with high sugar levels and could possibly face a diabetic or pre-diabetic diagnosis is because it runs in my family. In my career in the healthcare field, I have also seen the devastating effects that diabetes has on our community and the healthcare system. Remember when I went to the nutritionist, she was expecting a larger lady. My eyes were opened to the fact that there must be others who may not even realize how desperately they need to change.

Through my journey there were some challenges. For example, I saw an allergist and shared how mad I was that my HbA1c had stabilized for the past 12 months. You know everyone was in my ear; "If your sugar level is the same, you may as well go back and eat sugar." He quickly shut me down as he explained that if I had not given up sugar, I would be diabetic today. The signs were already there as far as the HbA1c levels going up and ultimately with the pre-diabetic diagnosis. Thus, had I continued to eat the way I was eating my body wouldn't have been able to handle it any longer. I did the right thing at the right time by eliminating sugar.

Someone recently told me that she knows a lady who has been totally sugar-free for 20 years. This is my goal. While I am not totally sugar free, I can say that I live sugar free, because sugar no longer has a hold on me. It once had a grip that was stronger than I knew, but through my changes I was just scratching the surface.

I rarely eat any sweets today. If I were to eat something sweet, I would just have a bite. I enjoy a bite and keep moving, because at this point things are too sweet and the cravings are gone. I know you are saying, "This could never be me". Believe me when I say, five years ago, I would have never imagined saying this either. Once you decide, and remain consistent, you won't go beyond the limits you set. This is especially true if you measure and make better choices.

Step 1: Decide
Step 2: Seek Help
Step 3: Research and Gradual Replacement
Step 4: Measure: *The most critical part of my process*

- I measured my blood glucose level to determine what foods I could eat and in what quantities.
- Someone can suggest what to eat. But by measuring your glucose levels; first thing in the morning, just before and two hours after you eat and before you go to bed. You get a picture of how **your** body reacts to what you are ingesting.

Evidence based personalized preventive medicine.

- I use measurement to change behavior; if my sugar level is high in the morning, I will choose tea in the morning instead of a cappuccino.
- I have eliminated wine because through measurement I found it affected my blood glucose levels in the morning.

Are you willing to measure to make a change?

Track your glucose levels, what trend are you seeing?

	Day 1	Day 2	Day 3	Day 4	Day 5
Morning					
2 Hours After Breakfast					
Lunch					
2 Hours After Lunch					
Dinner					
2 Hours After Dinner					
Bedtime					

CHAPTER 7

The Struggle is Real

Living sugar free is very much a struggle. The first year was especially challenging but I was successful in only eating five chocolate-covered strawberries on Valentine's Day, two Pepsi's and a piece of cake. I was scared straight!

Preparation is the key! In the beginning of every week, I make boiled eggs and put them in bags so that I could just grab them every morning. I also pre-pack snack bags of mixed nuts and cashews and have them at work, in the car and in my purse. Most of the "Kind" bars have six to seven grams of protein and five grams of sugar. By making intentional good choices, you can remain in control of your health each day. (Appendix 4 outlines other five grams of sugar or less snacks).

For my morning routine, I have five boiled egg whites and a cappuccino, mostly milk and sweetened with Stevia. After my cappuccino, I drink a sparkling water (I find that Le Croix has the best flavor). Drinking five to six glasses of water a day keeps me full, reduces my cravings and flushes the caffeine out of my system as well. Drinking this much water does get monotonous. So, I keep gum on hand to suppress cravings for sweets.

The strategy is carbohydrate reduction: My lunch is either soup or a salad; soup and a sandwich; or a hot meal. I try to reduce my carbohydrates by having chicken salad over a bed of spinach with melted provolone cheese and Baked Lay's Potato Chips.

For dinner, I have eliminated white carbohydrates. I usually have a protein (chicken or fish) and veggies! There are still carbs in my system because I haven't eliminated everything, but I have found ways to enjoy them wisely. There are ways to get carbs, even the ones that you love, and still make better choices for your overall health.

While traveling, do not be afraid to ask for what you want or need. On a recent flight to London, I left the house at 5:37 a.m., arrived and parked at the airport at 6:40 a.m. and began my trek to my gate. You know as well as I do that some airports are easier than others to traverse and Dulles International is a beast! By the time I got to the gate, there was no time for breakfast but thankfully, I was able to grab a 32 oz bottle of water and salt and pepper cashews. I stopped at two branches of Starbucks, but the lines were too long, and I was afraid of missing my flight. As soon as we boarded, I ate my cashews. About thirty minutes later, breakfast was served. The options were cinnamon toast or Tuscan omelet. Shocker, I chose the omelet. It came hot with potatoes along with a yogurt, cinnamon roll, pineapple and grapes. Since the flight is seven hours, I ate a few of the potatoes as well. Guess what? It did not fill me up. Instead of loading up on the carbs, high glycemic index fruit and yogurt, I simply asked at the end of the service if they would mind giving me a second omelet. At the end of the meal, while others enjoyed salted caramel gelato, I had a mini chocolate "Kind" bars. My dessert was only five grams of sugar vs. theirs with, what I imagine would be 20-30 grams of sugar. I followed this with gum to continue the flavor party. Of course, I continued to drink water as well to stay hydrated and remain full to decrease cravings.

During that trip, I also asked the course organizer ahead of time if we would be able to have protein options at the breaks during the class I was attending. More times than not, people will accommodate if you ask.

When I travel, I make sure that breakfast is my biggest meal of my day, so I do not easily get hungry. For dessert during business dinners, I either order berries or have a spoonful of a friend's dessert. On my first year of being sugar free, I would have abstained but now that I know what a whole slice of cake or pie will do to my sugar level, I can enjoy a bite. Knowing how my body reacts via the glucose monitoring changed my behavior by understanding the driver of my increased blood sugar level. You do better when you take time to know about the nutritional data of the food that you eat.

My pantry and refrigerator have nuts, Kind bars, plenty of kiwi and berries; black berries, strawberries and raspberries, and individually wrapped cheese for snacks or dessert. These, as well as apples, make great healthier dessert options. I also ensure that there is always sparkling water and unsweetened iced tea in the refrigerator.

Routine and preparation is all very well and good, but you may ask: what do I do if I cannot control the situation, especially if I am traveling or have whole day meetings? In this case, I bring my snack bags of mixed nuts and cashews, my sparkling water for flavor and I always make sure that I have my Stevia packets to sweeten tea if available. If I do not have nuts, I have Kind bars to ensure that I have a snack with at least five to six grams of protein with five grams of sugar or less. If there are times when the urge to eat sweets is strong, I eat my chocolate-covered almonds around 2 p.m. in the afternoon, early enough for my body to break it down.

Gum is also my friend, when I am looking for something in the afternoon, I eat gum to get a quick pop of flavor and sweetness. I always have gum on me: in my purse, my car, my desk drawer at work and even in my jacket pockets during meetings. I chew it long enough to get that pop of flavor, then I throw it away. The other trick I have at home is eating "Gummy Vitamins." They only have three to five grams of sugar. I pop them in my mouth after a meal; calcium and a multivitamin, again for flavor and a bit of sweetness to get me through the evening. I can see you rolling your eyes! You just have to try it. You will see that after you have kicked the sugar habit these small pops of sweetness will be all you need.

Don't get me wrong, I struggle with this every day. My current company provides free sodas and sparkling water. I am a Pepsi girl and there are plenty of days when I pray that there is not a diet Pepsi in the refrigerator at work. I say "Lord if there is a diet Pepsi in here it is meant for me!" Most other days - He makes it so there is only sparkling water in the refrigerator. Lately the fridge is stocked, so it helps that I have unsweetened iced tea as an alternative. Most days this works, but on days when I am stressed or tired, I have a diet Pepsi and keep moving. I used to say if 80 percent of the time I am doing the right thing (eat well during the week) and 20 percent of the time (eat what I want on weekends) worked for me.

Now, I know my body cannot handle this and I have to prepare and make better choices. I have truly made a lifestyle change.

A few of my aunts have struggled with heart disease and diabetes. The link has been proven to exist between diabetes and cardiovascular diseases. I have seen them struggle personally and I am determined to use their struggle as a motivation to overcome my own. I was able to sustain being sugar free by staying balanced, not cutting any essential nutrients out but not having as much carbs as I used to. Keeping even the smallest of changes, like not eating corn and not putting syrup on my pancakes, has been very important along with regular exercise.

My dad is 93 and my mom's cousin is 105 years old. I am determined to live longer in my retired years than my working years because of the longevity in my family – I want those years to be healthy! That is why I tell myself that "I can get through this" every time, every day that I struggle. If you mess up – recommit! Let yesterday go, today's a new day, recommit today!

CHAPTER 8

Step #5: Recommit and Move; This is What Success Looks Like

Those are the four steps for me that led to my success. When I say success, I mean progress. When you are making progress, you are succeeding. I am still on this journey and I want to coach you as you begin your journey. The time and dedication I've put into this has given me a head start and the knowledge to help you begin Sugar Free Living and stop the progression to becoming diabetic. I would love to be your coach and assist you through this exhilarating adventure.

I know that it can be hard and may seem impossible. It was hard for me, but it is possible. Having a coach on your side who has been through the battles makes it a little easier. Right now, I live with cookies and candy in my pantry and I don't give in to the temptation. I just make different choices than I used to make. Another key is being prepared with alternatives. I now have cocoa almonds, both at home and work, take boiled egg whites with me on my way into work to eat protein with my cappuccino and always have berries or apples around for a dessert.

I had to work up to this and constantly am measuring my glucose levels and evaluating my decisions based on my sugar level.

My results are proof that you can succeed if you are willing to put in the necessary discipline. Here are the results of my lifestyle changes.
- **After 2.5 years, I am no longer pre-diabetic**
- I reduced my HbA1c by 10%
- I have sustained a 11.5 % reduction in my weight over three years
- I went from a women's size "8" to a size "0"
- For the first time in my adult life, I have a flat stomach after three children

There are still daily struggles and tough choices that must be made. During the first year, I said, "No" to chocolate in Switzerland, but had sugar free ice cream at the end of the school year to celebrate with my kids. I ate sugar free chocolates the first six months, but now I don't eat anything with a chemical sweetener. The phased approach and working with a nutritionist helped but measurement was the key. The constant feedback from measuring my glucose level is a daily reminder of what I want and don't want and is how I stay on track and focused on my health. This daily measurement does not have to be a chore. I have a glucometer in my purse, to take levels during the day, and one that I keep in my bathroom to take my morning and evening readings.

When making the decision that I did not want to live with diabetes and that I wanted to share my life with my husband and my family; changes had to be made. Living life from a wheelchair is not an option for me. I am not ready to just coast along in life hoping to see the world, while losing my eyesight because of a problem I ignored. I want to experience life with my family from a position of choice, health and wholeness. I certainly do not want any prognosis that includes heart issues.

According to the National Institute of Diabetes and Digestive and Kidney Diseases (NIDDK), "having diabetes means that you are more likely to develop heart disease and have a greater chance of a heart attack or a stroke." You will find the NIDDK website clearly shows the link between diabetes, heart disease, and stroke. It goes on to state, "Over time, high blood glucose from diabetes can damage your blood vessels and the nerves that control your heart and blood vessels. The longer you have diabetes, the higher the chances that you will develop heart disease."

This meant changing my diet would not be enough. A final step would be required of me if my goals are to be realized. A consistent 150 minutes of exercise a week and at least 10k steps per day is my current goal. During this journey, I have exercised; but have not made a consistent effort. How could I make so many sacrifices and not put forth the effort to exercise? It seemed like common sense to me and the payoff would be well worth the cost. My daughter has a 13-year-old diabetic friend and shared that if her blood sugar was 200 and she played tennis, it would come down to 120. I have recommitted to my health, daily and weekly! Sometimes it is decision by decision as we are conscious about our choices.

Success in this journey is not a destination, but rather a continual progression towards better living. Sometimes there are high points and sometimes there are low points. Eliminating bit by bit was necessary in the beginning. Now if I occasionally want a spoonful of ice cream or a fork full of cake, I have a taste and move on! I'm satisfied with a sample and frankly I now find them too sweet!

It took three years to go from eliminating a little to winning most battles over cravings. Now I prepare in advance and anticipate my needs before the cravings or hunger pains arise.

I always have boiled eggs in the refrigerator, I bring five grams or less snacks to work (cinnamon covered pumpkin seeds or cocoa covered almonds). I'm prepared when I must satisfy cravings during "that time of the month" and to get over the 2 p.m. mid-day hump). I even bring sparkling water to meetings to bring flavor into my life.

You see, there is always room for improvement. There are people we deemed perfect and are recognized. Unfortunately the recognition is often temporary; for example the title of "Sexiest Man Alive. "It is rare if anyone holds the title for more than a single year. Therefore, finding ways to constantly improve your health is success. Making changes in your diet is doable! Commit to these **FIVE** simple steps.

Today there is no cure for Type 1 diabetes. You have the POWER to choose a healthy life free of diabetes. If you are reading this book, like me, you believe in self-investment! This is your time to get the support you need to succeed.

I see a world without diabetes and it starts with your sugar free living. As your lifestyle coach, I have your success formula; will hold you accountable, help you avoid pitfalls and help navigate you to a healthy abundant life.

Step 1: Decide

Step 2: Seek Help

Step 3: Research and Gradual Replacement

Step 4: Measure

Step 5: Recommit and Move

- This is a marathon... not a sprint: Eliminate sugar, reduce carbohydrate intake and measure your glucose levels.
- Find ways to bring movement and exercise into your life: Set a goal of 150 minutes per week.
- Recommit to your health goals; it's a daily struggle with hourly choices.
- Reclaim your Why and Celebrate your Success.

Are you willing to make the necessary commitment to change your life?

YOU'RE JUST FIVE STEPS AWAY FROM A SUGAR-FREE LIFE:

1. Decide

2. Seek Help

3. Research and Gradual Replacement

4. Measure

5. Recommit and Move

It's Oh, So Sweet to Live Sugar Free!

Alcoholic Beverages with 5 Grams of Sugar or Less

Get your Drink On!

Item		Sugar
1.	Spiked Seltzer	5g
2.	Truly Spiked & Sparkling Wild Berry Hard Soda	1g
3.	Smirnoff Sparkling Seltzer Spiked	0g
4.	White Claw Hard Seltzer	4g
5.	Henry's Hard Sparkling Water	0g
6.	Nauti Seltzer Hard Seltzer	0g

Glycemic Index (GI)

Know the Numbers

BREAKFAST CEREAL

Low GI

All-Bran (UK/Aus)	30
All-Bran (US)	50
Oat Bran	50
Rolled Oats	51
Special K (UK/Aus)	54
Natural Muesli	40
Porridge	58

Medium GI

Bran Buds	58
Mini Wheats	58
Nutri-Grain	66
Shredded Wheat	67
Porridge Oats	63
Special K (US)	69

High GI

Cornflakes	80
Sultana Bran	73
Bran Flakes	74
Coco Pops	77
Puffed Wheat	80
Oats in Honey Bake	77
Team	82
Total	76
Cheerios	74
Rice Krispies	82
Weetabix	74

STAPLES

Low GI

Wheat Pasta Shapes	54
New Potatoes	54
Meat Ravioli	39
Spaghetti	32
Tortellini (Cheese)	50
Egg Fettuccini	32
Brown Rice	50
Buckwheat	51
White Long Grain Rice	50
Pearled Barley	22
Yam	35
Sweet Potatoes	48
Instant Noodles	47
Wheat Tortilla	30

Medium GI

Basmati Rice	58
Couscous	61
Cornmeal	68
Taco Shells	68
Gnocchi	68
Canned Potatoes	61
Chinese (Rice) Vermicelli	58
Baked Potatoes	60
Wild Rice	57

High GI

Instant White Rice	87
Glutinous Rice	86
Short Grain White Rice	83
Tapioca	70
Fresh Mashed Potatoes	73
French Fries	75
Instant Mashed Potatoes	80

BREAD

Low GI

Soya and Linseed	36
Wholegrain Pumpernickel	46
Heavy Mixed Grain	45
Whole Wheat	49
Sourdough Rye	48
Sourdough Wheat	54

Medium GI

Croissant	67
Hamburger Bun	61
Pita, White	57
Whole Meal Rye	62

High GI

White	71
Bagel	72
French Baguette	95

DAIRY

Low GI

Whole Milk	31
Skimmed Milk	32
Chocolate Milk	42
Sweetened Yogurt	33
Artificially Sweetened Yogurt	23
Custard	35
Soy Milk	44

Medium GI

Ice Cream	62

VEGETABLES

Low GI

Frozen Green Peas	39
Frozen Sweet Corn	47
Raw Carrots	16
Boiled Carrots	41
Eggplant	15
Broccoli	10
Cauliflower	15
Cabbage	10
Mushrooms	10
Tomatoes	15
Chilies	10
Lettuce	10
Green Beans	15
Red Peppers	10
Onions	10

Medium GI

Beetroot	64

High GI

Pumpkin	75
Parsnips	97

LEGUMES (Beans)

Low GI

Kidney Beans (canned)	52
Butter Beans	36
Chick Peas	42
Haricot/Navy Beans	31
Lentils, Red	21
Lentils, Green	30
Pinto Beans	45
Black-Eyed Beans	50
Yellow Split Peas	32

Medium GI

Beans in Tomato Sauce	56

FRUITS

Low GI

Cherries	22
Plums	24
Grapefruit	25
Peaches	28
Peach, Canned in Natural Juice	30
Apples	34
Pears	41
Dried Apricots	32
Grapes	43
Coconut	45
Coconut Milk	41
Kiwi Fruit	47
Oranges	40
Strawberries	40
Prunes	29

Medium GI

Mango	60
Sultanas	56
Bananas	58
Raisins	64
Papaya	60
Figs	61
Pineapple	66

High GI

Watermelon	80
Dates	103

SNACKS & SWEET FOODS

Low GI

Slim-Fast Meal Replacement	27
Snickers Bar (high fat)	41
Nut & Seed Muesli Bar	49
Sponge Cake	46
Nutella	33
Milk Chocolate	42
Hummus	6
Peanuts	13
Walnuts	15
Cashew Nuts	25
Nuts and Raisins	21
Jam	51
Corn Chips	42
Oatmeal Crackers	55

Medium GI

Ryvita	63
Digestives	59
Blueberry Muffin	59
Honey	58

High GI

Pretzels	83
Water Crackers	78
Rice Cakes	87
Puffed Crispbread	81
Donuts	76
Scones	92
Maple Flavored Syrup	68

The glycemic index range is as follows:

Low GI = 55 or less **Medium GI** = 56 - 69 **High GI** = 70 or more

Diabetes 101

Start Your Research

When I researched, I not only learned about glycemic index, I also had to educate myself with the language of diabetes. This section outlines key terms you will hear from your doctor.

Diabetes mellitus **type 2** (also known as **type 2 diabetes**) is a long-term metabolic disorder that is characterized by high blood sugar, insulin resistance, and relative lack of insulin. Common symptoms include increased thirst, frequent urination, and unexplained weight loss. **Type 2 Diabetes** (T2D) is more common than type 1 diabetes with about 90 to 95 percent of people with diabetes having T2D.[ii]

Endocrinologists are doctors who specialize in glands and the hormones they make. They deal with metabolism, or all the biochemical processes that make your body work, including how your body changes food into energy and how it grows. They may work with adults or kids.[iii]

Gestational diabetes is a condition in which a woman without diabetes develops high blood sugar levels during pregnancy. Long term, children are at higher risk of being overweight and developing type 2 diabetes. Gestational diabetes is caused by not enough insulin in the setting of insulin resistance.[iv]

A **glucometer**, also known as a glucose meter or blood glucose monitoring device, is a home measurement system you can use to test the amount of glucose (sugar) in your blood.[v]

Glucose: The simple sugar that is the chief source of energy. Glucose is found in the blood and is the main sugar that the body manufactures. The body makes glucose from all three elements of food 'protein, fats, and carbohydrates 'but the largest amount of glucose derives from carbohydrates. Glucose serves as the major source of energy for living cells. However, cells cannot use glucose without the help of insulin. Also known as dextrose.[vi]

The **Glycemic Index** (GI) is a relative ranking of carbohydrate in foods according to how they affect blood glucose levels. Carbohydrates with a low GI value (55 or less) are more slowly digested, absorbed and metabolized and cause a lower and slower rise in blood glucose and, therefore usually, insulin levels.[vii]

A **hemoglobin A1c (HbA1c)** test measures the amount of blood sugar (glucose) attached to hemoglobin. Hemoglobin is the part of your red blood cells that carries oxygen from your lungs to the rest of your body. An HbA1c test shows what the average amount of glucose attached to hemoglobin has been over the past three months. It's a three-month average because that's typically how long a red blood cell lives.

For people without diabetes:
- The normal range for the HbA1c level is between 4% and 5.6%.
- HbA1c levels between 5.7% and 6.4% means you have a higher chance of getting diabetes.
- Levels of 6.5% or higher means you have diabetes. [viii]

Hypoglycemia: Low blood sugar (glucose). Hypoglycemia may be associated with symptoms such as anxiety, sweating, tremor, palpitations, nausea, and pallor. Hypoglycemia also starves the brain of glucose energy, which is essential for proper brain function. Lack of glucose energy to the brain can cause symptoms ranging from headache, mild confusion, abnormal behavior, loss of consciousness, seizure, and coma.[ix]

Insulin resistance occurs when the body doesn't respond as well to the insulin that the pancreas is making, and glucose is less able to enter the cells. People with insulin resistance may or may not go on to develop Type 2 Diabetes.[x]

Metabolic Syndrome is a cluster of conditions (increased blood pressure, high blood sugar, excess body fat around the waist, and abnormal cholesterol or triglyceride levels) that occur together, increasing your risk of heart disease, stroke and diabetes.[xi]

Pre-diabetes is an indication that you could develop type 2 Diabetes if you don't make some lifestyle changes. It is a condition characterized by slightly elevated blood glucose levels, regarded as indicative that a person is at risk of progressing to type 2 diabetes.[xii]

Type 1 Diabetes, once known as **juvenile diabetes** or **insulin-dependent diabetes**, is a chronic condition in which the pancreas produces little or no insulin. Insulin is a hormone needed to allow sugar (glucose) to enter cells to produce energy. [xiii]

Pre-diabetes is a "pre-diagnosis" of diabetes—you can think of it as a warning sign. It's when your blood glucose level (blood sugar level) is higher than normal, but it's not high enough to be considered diabetes.[xiv]

Snacks with 6 Grams of Sugar or Less

Start Munching! Eat This!

Item		Serving	Sugar	Protein
1.	Kind Cashew & Ginger Spice Bar	1 bar	4g	6g
2.	Kind Dark Chocolate Cinnamon Pecan Bar	1 bar	5g	4g
3.	Kind Madagascar Vanilla Almond Bar	1 bar	4g	6g
4.	Kind Dark Chocolate Nuts & Sea Salt Bar	1 bar	5g	6g
5.	Kettle Popcorn	2 cups	2g	6g
6.	Blue Diamond Almonds Coffee Caramel Macchiato Almonds	24 nuts	3g	6g
7.	The Good Bean Sweet Cinnamon Roasted Chickpea Snacks	1/8 cup	6g	5g
8.	Health Warrior Chia Bars, Coconut	1 bar	4g	3g
9.	Somersault Snack Co. Crunchy Nuggets Dutch Cocoa	14 pieces	4g	6g
10.	Planters Dark Chocolate flavor Cocoa Almonds	24 pieces	4g	6g
11.	P3 Portal Protein Packs and Deli Snackers		<4g	5-15g

Naturally Flavored Beverages with 5 Grams of Sugar or Less

Get your Drink On!

Item	Sugar
1. Hint Fruit Infused Water:	5g
2. Bai Flavored Water Antioxidant Infused	1g
3. SoBe Water	0g
4. Capri Sun Roarin' Waters Flavored	0g
5. Core Organic Water	0g
6. Pure Leaf, Brewed Unsweet Tea	0g
7. Core Hydration Water	0g
8. Perrier Carbonated Mineral Water	0g
9. San Pellegrino Sparkling Natural Mineral Water	0g
10. La Croix Sparkling Waters	0g
11. Spindrift Flavor Water	0g
12. Sparkling Ice Sparkling Water	0g
13. Glaceau Vitamin Water Zero	0g
14. Stur Liquid Water Enhancer	0g

ABOUT THE AUTHOR

Kathy "Sugar Free Girl" Williams; has a passion for people and a mission to prevent diabetes in 1M people. As a Diabetes Prevention Specialist, she has created the Power Academy and Health Investment Institute which are 12-month group coaching programs designed to stop the progression of diabetes in people diagnosed with gestational or pre-diabetes.

She helps shift your mindset about sugar, prevent disease and sustain results so you can live an abundant life. She can help you overcome your biggest challenges and stop the dieting cycle with this lifestyle change.

Her vision of a diabetes-free world was the result of her own journey from a pre-diabetic diagnosis to complete wellness. She is eager to share her learnings which led her to phenomenal results:
- No longer pre-diabetic
- Reduced HbA1c by 10%
- Dropped 4 dress sizes
- Sustained an 11% weight reduction

Highly qualified to offer health information, Kathy is a Marketing Director at a biotechnology company and has been in the healthcare industry for more than 20 years. She has worked as an Engineer, Brand Manager, and New Business Development Manager in the Medical Device, Pharmaceutical, Vaccines, and Clinical Diagnostics markets.

Kathy has a Master's in Business Administration and Strategy from the Goizueta School of Business, a Master of Science degree in Mechanical Engineering from the University of Cincinnati and a Bachelor of Science degree from North Carolina A&T State University. She also holds a certification from the University of Pittsburgh's Diabetes Prevention Program's (DPP) Group Lifestyle Balance™ Coach Training Program.

Sugar Free Living Changed her life. It can change yours too!

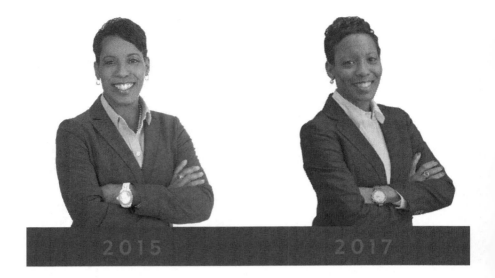

Connect with Kathy!
Let's schedule a strategy session to discuss your health goals and let's build your new healthy abundant life. Reach out to me at **Kathy@ilivesugarfree.com**.

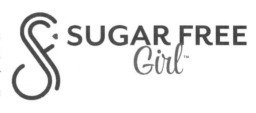

I would love to hear how my journey impacted your life. Join my FREE Facebook community (Sugar Free Nation with Sugar Free Girl) where I share sugar free living and other health tips. I'm here for you!

---

i   www.cdc.gov/media/releases/2014/p0610-diabetes-report.html
ii   en.wikipedia.org/wiki/Diabetes_mellitus_type_2
iii www.webmd.com/diabetes/what-is-endocrinologist#1
iv   en.wikipedia.org/wiki/Gestational_diabetes
v   en.wikipedia.org/wiki/Glucose_meter
vi   www.medicinenet.com/script/main/art.asp?articlekey=3608
vii www.gisymbol.com/about-glycemic-index
viii medlineplus.gov/lab-tests/hemoglobin-a1c-hba1c-test/
ix   www.medicinenet.com/script/main/art.asp?articlekey=3856
x   kidshealth.org/en/parents/insulin-resistance.html
xi   www.mayoclinic.org/diseases-conditions/metabolic-syndrome/symptoms-causes/syc-20351916
xii www.endocrineweb.com/conditions/pre-diabetes/pre-diabetes
xiii www.mayoclinic.org/diseases-conditions/type-1-diabetes/symptoms-causes/syc-20353011
xiv www.endocrineweb.com/conditions/pre-diabetes/pre-diabetes

Made in the USA
Middletown, DE
01 August 2020